Nutrition yoga benefits

BY : George Mantar

Table of Contents

1

EATING, AN ACT THAT CONCERNS THE TOTALITY OF BEING

What I will tell you about nutrition is of the utmost importance, my dear brothers and sisters, and very few people, even the most educated and advanced, know about it. First of all, of course, you will find that it is not so interesting, but by listening to me, and above all by beginning to put these truths into practice, you will be compelled to recognize that they can enrich, beautify and transform your existence.

Suppose that as a result of certain circumstances you have been deprived of food for several days: you are so weak that you can no longer walk or make a single movement. Even if you are extremely educated or wealthy, all your knowledge and possessions are worth nothing compared to a piece of bread or a piece of fruit that someone brings you. At the first bite, you already feel revived. Isn't that wonderful? This single bite has activated so many mechanisms and forces that an entire existence could not suffice to enumerate them all.

But have you ever stopped to think about the power of the elements contained in food and the fact that, to get you back on your feet, a meal will always be more effective than your thoughts, your feelings or your will?... This food to which you attach only instinctive importance, and not an intellectual, conscious importance, it is she and she alone who is able to restore your energy and health. Thanks to it, you can continue to act, to speak, to feel, to think.

Among their work, the Initiates have given great importance to research on nutrition. They have found that the food, which is prepared in the divine laboratories with inexpressible wisdom, contains the magic elements capable of preserving or restoring not only physical but psychic health and of bringing about the greatest revelations. But to benefit from these elements, it is necessary to know the conditions to be fulfilled.

Obviously, we cannot fail to see that the whole world puts the question of food in the first place. Everyone tries first to settle this question, they work every day and even fight for it - many wars and revolutions have no other origin! But this attitude towards food is still only an instinct that humans have in common with animals; they have not yet understood the spiritual importance of the act of eating, they do not know how to eat. Observe them during a meal: they take in food mechanically, unconsciously, they swallow without chewing, they stir up chaotic thoughts and feelings in their heads and hearts, and often even argue while eating. This is how they disrupt the functioning of their organism:

Thousands of people get sick without knowing that their illnesses come from the way they eat. You just have to see what happens in families: before the meal, no one has anything to say to each other, everyone is busy in their corner reading, listening to the radio or doing tinkering... But when it comes to sitting down to table, everyone has stories to tell or even scores to settle, and they talk, they argue, they bicker. After such a meal you have to go to rest or even sleep, because you feel drowsy, heavy, and those who have to work do it without taste or enthusiasm. While the one who knew how to eat correctly is lucid and well disposed.

You will say: "But then, how should one eat?..." I will speak to you about the way an Initiate conceives of nutrition. As it is for him to put himself in the best conditions to receive the elements prepared in the laboratories of nature, an Initiate begins by recollecting himself by binding himself to the Creator, and above all he does not launch into conversations, he eat in silence.

Silence during meals should not be regarded merely as a convent habit; a sage, an Initiate eats in silence. And when he takes the first bite he tries to chew it consciously, as long as possible, until it disappears in his mouth without him even having to swallow it. Because the state in which you take the first bite is extremely important. It is therefore necessary to prepare to do so in the best possible dispositions, because it is this first bite that internally triggers all the cogs. Never forget that the most important moment of an act is its beginning, it is he who gives the signal for the release of the forces, and these forces do not stop on the way, they go until the end. If you start in a harmonious state,

You have to eat slowly and chew well, because that helps digestion, of course, but also for another reason: the mouth, which is the first to receive food, is the most important laboratory, because the more spiritual. The mouth plays on a more subtle level the role of a real stomach; it absorbs the etheric particles of food, the finer and more powerful energies, and it is the gross materials which are then sent into the stomach.

The mouth contains extremely sophisticated apparatus, glands located on the tongue and under the tongue, which have the task of capturing the etheric particles of food. How many times have you had this experience! You were there, hungry, almost lifeless, and you started to eat... From the first mouthfuls, even before the food could be digested, you already felt restored, invigorated. How could this have happened so quickly? Thanks to the mouth, the organism has already absorbed energies, etheric elements which went to feed the nervous system. Before the stomach receives food, the nervous system is already nourished.

When I speak of the etheric elements to be sought from food, you should not be surprised. A fruit, for example, is made of solid, liquid, gaseous, etheric matter. Everyone is familiar with solids and liquids. Much less concern themselves with perfumes which are already more subtle and which belong to the domain of the air. As for the etheric side which is linked to the colors of the fruit and especially to its life, it is a totally ignored and neglected area, but which is nevertheless of the greatest importance, because it is thanks to the etheric particles of food that the man nourishes his subtle bodies.

Since man does not only have a physical body but other more subtle bodies, the seats of his psychic and spiritual functions (etheric, astral, mental, causal, Buddhist, atmic body), the question arises precisely for him to know how to nourish these subtle bodies which, because of one's ignorance, often remain without nourishment. He knows roughly what he should give to his physical body (I say: roughly, because most humans eat meat, which is harmful to their physical and mental health), but he does not know feed the other bodies: the etheric body (or vital body), the astral body (seat of feelings and emotions), the mental body (seat of the intellect), and even less the other superior bodies.

I told you that you have to chew food well, but chewing is above all for the physical body. For the etheric body we must add the breath. Just as air kindles a flame - you know you have to blow on a fire to rekindle it - so deep breaths during a meal produce better combustion. Digestion is only combustion, just like respiration and reflection; only the degree of heat and the purity of the material differ from process to process. So, while eating, you have to stop from time to time and breathe deeply, so that this combustion allows the etheric body to draw more subtle particles from the food. The etheric body being the carrier of vitality, memory and sensitivity, you benefit from its proper development.

The astral body, on the other hand, feeds on feelings, on emotions, therefore on elements which are made of an even finer material than etheric particles. By stopping for a few moments with love on food, you prepare your astral body to extract from it particles more precious than etheric particles. When the astral body has absorbed these elements, it has every possibility of arousing feelings of an extremely high order: love for the whole world, the feeling of being happy, at peace and of living in harmony with Nature.

Unfortunately, humans are increasingly losing this feeling: they no longer feel this protection, this solicitude, this love, this friendship of objects, trees, mountains, stars; they are worried, disturbed, and even when they are at home in the shelter, even during their sleep, they have the impression of being threatened. It is a subjective impression, because in reality they are not so much threatened, but inside something is crumbling and they no longer feel protected by Mother Nature because their astral body has not received its nourishment.

Feed your astral body and you will experience indescribable feelings of well-being that will push you to manifest yourselves with generosity and benevolence. If you have to settle important issues, you will know how to be broad, understanding and make concessions.

To nourish his mental body, an Initiate concentrates on food, and he even closes his eyes to concentrate better. Since food represents for him a manifestation of the Divinity, he strives to study it in all its aspects: where it comes from, what it contains, what qualities correspond to it, what entities have of it, because invisible beings work on each tree, on each plant. His mind absorbed in these reflections, he draws nourishment from the elements superior to the elements of the astral plane. From there is born for him a clarity, a deep penetration of life and the world. After a meal taken in such conditions, he rises from the table with such luminous understanding that he is capable of undertaking the greatest works of thought.

Most people think that reading, studying and thinking are enough to develop their intellectual capacities. No, study and reflection are essential but insufficient activities; during meals the mental body must also be nourished in order to become resistant and susceptible to prolonged effort.

It must be understood that the astral and mental bodies being the supports, one of feeling, the other of thought, these two bodies need to receive appropriate nourishment so that man can assume his task in the affective domains. and intellectual.

Beyond the etheric, astral and mental bodies, man has other bodies of an even more spiritual essence: the causal, buddhic and atmic bodies, seats of reason, soul and spirit, who also need to be fed. You will nurture them by allowing yourself to be filled with a feeling of gratitude towards the Creator. This feeling of gratitude, which humans are also losing more and more, will open to you the heavenly doors through which you will receive the greatest blessings. At that moment everything will unfold before you and you will see, you will feel, you will live! Gratitude is capable of transforming coarse matter into light, into joy, and one must learn to use it.

If you know how to feed your three superior bodies, the subtle particles which you will have thus captured will be distributed everywhere, in the brain, in the solar plexus, in all the organs. You will begin to realize that you have other needs, other joys, of a higher nature, and greater possibilities will also open up to you.

When you have finished eating, you should not get up right away to start work or discussions. But it is also not good to go and spend an hour or two in an armchair or a chaise longue. If you lie down to rest, supposedly, in reality you don't rest, you become heavy, your organism becomes sluggish. When you have finished eating, remain quiet for a moment by taking a few deep breaths which will allow a better distribution of energies in the body; you will then feel extremely well disposed to undertake all kinds of work.

It is not enough to start the meal well, you must also finish it in the best possible way to give a good start to the different tasks that await you. Never forget that every activity has

its beginning and that this beginning
is the essential moment.

2

HRANI-YOGA

These days, people who are disoriented by a hectic life are looking for ways to regain their balance, and they are doing yoga, Zen, transcendental meditation, or they are going to learn how to relax. I'm not saying it's not a good thing, but I found a simpler and more effective exercise: learning to eat.

When you eat haphazardly, in noise, nervousness, haste, discussions, what's the point of then going to meditate or do yoga? What comedy! Why not understand that every day, two or three times a day, we all have the opportunity to do an exercise in relaxation, concentration, harmonization of all our cells?

If I ask you to make the effort to eat in silence (not only not to speak, but not to make any noise with the cutlery), chewing each bite for a long time, taking a few deep breaths from time to time, but especially concentrating on food and thanking Heaven for all this richness, it is that these exercises, so insignificant in appearance, are among the best for acquiring true self-mastery. It is mastering these little things that will give you the ability to master the big ones. When I see someone who is careless and clumsy in little things, it is easy for me to know not only how messy they have lived in the past, but how all of their deficiencies are going to reflect negatively on their future. Because everything is connected.

Obviously, it is difficult to be silent during meals to concentrate only on food... And if we manage to be silent and control our gestures externally, we make noise internally... Or, if we manage to to calm down inside, it is the thought which wanders elsewhere. This is why I tell you that nutrition is a yoga, because knowing how to eat requires attention, concentration, mastery.

But to be able to concentrate your thoughts during meals, you must have already acquired the habit of mastering it in everyday life. If you're always careful not to let negative thoughts and feelings overwhelm you, then yes, the groundwork is set, and it's easy. You will say: “But then, do you have to prepare all your life just to eat properly? " Yes and no...

Not all problems can be solved because one only knows how to eat properly. We take meals as a starting point, that does not mean that there is nothing more important and that all the rest of the day we can let ourselves go. Don't misunderstand me. It is all day long that one must be attentive and vigilant, and also maintain this attention and this vigilance during meals.

A meal is a magical ceremony through which food must be transformed into health, strength, love, light. Observe yourself: when you have eaten in a state of agitation, anger, revolt, it is all day afterwards that you manifest yourself with bitterness, nervousness, partiality, and if you have problems that are difficult to solve, the balance always tilts to the negative side. You then try to justify yourself by saying, "What do you want. Dude, I can't help it, I'm nervous," and to calm you down you take medicine, which isn't much use. To improve the state of your nervous system, learn to eat.

When you find yourself in front of food, you must leave everything aside, even the most important matters, because the most important thing is to eat according to the divine rules. If you have eaten correctly, the rest will settle very quickly. Eating correctly therefore saves a lot of time and saves a lot of energy. Do not imagine that you can solve problems more easily and quickly by being in a state of feverishness and tension; instead, you drop things from your hands, say awkward words, jostle people, and then have to spend whole days fixing the mess.

Most humans don't see that the smallest activities of daily living are of great significance, so how can they be made to understand that meals can be an opportunity for them to develop their intelligence, their love and their will? Intelligence, everyone thinks that it develops through study, or at least through difficulties and trials (when you are in trouble, a faculty finally awakens which pushes you to reflect and find the way out)... The heart, when you have a wife, children that you have to protect, help. Here, during meals, the heart? Do you think!... And the will, when one makes physical efforts, sports, etc. No, those who reason like this haven't understood anything yet.

It is during meals that you must begin to take care of the essentials, that is to say, to develop your heart, your intellect and your will. Yes, because it is never certain that everyone can go to libraries or university, that they have a wife and children, or that they find so many opportunities to exercise. But to eat, all are obliged to eat.

So take a look: do you want to develop your intellect? Well, you have the opportunity whenever you want to use the objects that are on the table. Try to pick them up and put them down without bumping into them, without jostling anything nearby, this is a good exercise in attention, in foresight. When I see how people knock their cutlery or drop it, I already know the flaws in their intelligence. They may have graduated from several universities, but I find that they still have major intellectual gaps. But yes, what use are diplomas if you don't yet know how to assess distances?

We want, suppose, to move a glass, but we have not seen how far it was, in front or behind another object, and knock! we hit him. It's a very small detail, but it reveals a flaw that will manifest in a much bigger way in life. These little clumsiness during meals announce that, in everyday life, some will do a lot of damage. They are the clue that they lack a certain interior attention, and we can already see on a small scale what they will do in the important events of existence: how they will speak and act without attention, jostling others , bumping into them, and they will take years to fix their gaffes and suffer.

Look, when I take this bottle out of the fridge, before I use it I have to think it's wet and if I don't wipe it, it can slip out of my hands and break the glass or the plate . So I have to wipe it if I want to grab it and be sure it won't escape me. It is the same for everything, at the table and in life... If an object escapes your vision, your consciousness, you are no longer its master and it does not obey you. To dominate an object, you must first dominate it in thought; if it escapes you, you will never be its master.

Before you sit down to eat, also try to see if anything is missing so that you don't have to get up several times during the meal to fetch a knife, a plate, some salt... It's something you I often observed when I was invited; twenty times the mistress of the house was obliged to get up because she had forgotten this, forgotten that... Yet we know very well what is needed since it is the same thing that is repeated every day. No, we don't even realize it, and all of life it goes on, all of life we forget and we have to interrupt meals to go get what we forgot. There is always something missing, and that is a sign that in other areas of life one is similarly inattentive and careless. So, how can we believe that we will be successful?

To develop your heart you will avoid making noise and disturbing others who also need to calm down, concentrate, meditate. Many think: “The others? but what can it do to me? And that's why the whole world is collapsing: because we don't think of others. Humans are unable to live together because they have no respect, no care for each other. Eating together is therefore a wonderful opportunity to develop and broaden one's consciousness.

The sign of a human being's evolution is his awareness of belonging to a much larger whole than himself, the harmony of which he takes care not to disturb through his activity, his thoughts, his feelings, his inner noise. You will say: “What, the internal noise? Yes, all noise is the result of dissonance, and the noise we make internally with our torments, our revolts, disturbs the psychic atmosphere. Whoever makes this noise does not know that, even for him, it is very bad, and that one day this noise will appear in his organism in the form of a psychic or even physical illness.

As you take the food, also remember to send your love to her, because that's when she opens up to give you all her treasures. Look at the flowers: when the sun warms them, they open, and when it disappears they close. And the food ? If you don't like it, it will give you almost nothing, it will close. But love it, eat it with love, it will open up and exhale its fragrance, it will give you all its etheric particles. You are used to eating automatically, without love, just to fill a void. But try to eat with love, you will see in what a wonderful state you will feel.

I know well that it is useless to speak of love to most humans, they do not know what love is: to greet with love, to walk with love, to speak with love, to look with love, to breathe with love, work with love... they don't know! Love, they believe, is only about being in bed with someone; no, precisely, that is not often love, and it shows! If they knew how to truly love, all of Heaven would be with them.

During meals you therefore develop your intellect and your heart, but also your will, since you get into the habit of controlling your gestures, of making them measured, harmonious... And the gesture is in the domain of the will. On days when you feel nervous, consider meals as an opportunity to learn how to calm yourself down; chew the food slowly, pay attention to your movements: a few minutes later, you will have regained your composure. There are very simple remedies for nervousness. You have started talking or working in agitation: if you do nothing, you will remain agitated all day and all your energies will go away because you forgot to "turn off the taps"... So stop - you for a minute, don't speak, don't move... then take another rhythm, another orientation.

It is during meals that we must begin to learn control, mastery. So, practice eating, watching your movements to make absolutely no noise. I know that what I am asking of you is almost the most impossible thing to do, but you will get there and everyone who comes here will be amazed. They will say, "But it's not possible, I can't believe my eyes!" And I'll say, "Well, at least believe your ears!" »

When you have eaten in silence and in peace, you then keep this state all day. Even if you have to run right and left, you only have to stop for a second to feel that peace is still there. Because you ate properly. Otherwise, whatever you do, rest, try to speak calmly, you are restless, confused, hectic.

From now on nutrition will be considered one of the best yogas that exist, although it has never been mentioned anywhere. All the other yogas: Radja-, Karma-, Hatha-, Jnana-, Kriya-, Agni-yogas are magnificent, but it takes years to obtain a small result. While with Hrani-yoga[1](that's what I call it), the results are very fast. It is the easiest, most accessible yoga; it is practiced by all creatures without exception, although still unconsciously. All the alchemy and magic is contained in this most misunderstood and misunderstood yoga to date.

This is why, even if you are overwhelmed with occupations, do not hide behind this pretext for having no spiritual life. Three times a day, at least, you have the best conditions to bind yourself to Heaven, to the Lord, since three times a day you are obliged to eat. Everyone is forced to eat. We don't have time to pray, we don't have time to read, to meditate, of course, but we are obliged to devote at least a few minutes to eating. So why not take advantage of this moment to perfect yourself, to bind yourself to the Lord, to send him a thought of gratitude and love?

From now on, let meals be an opportunity for you to do this spiritual work that is so essential. Many people think they are perfect because they conform to the laws of society: they do no harm to anyone, they conscientiously fulfill their professional and family duties. But in spite of that the divine world is closed for them, and they do not have this joy, this happiness, this plenitude, this light which the divine life brings. They think they are perfect, yes, but what perfection? Funny perfection where there is never time for the soul and for the spirit!

Of course, you have to work to support yourself and not be a burden to anyone, but you also have to find a few minutes to nourish the soul and the spirit. We came to earth with a great mission, but many forget it to think only of their social success, and they take themselves for models! But which models? No light comes from them, they have not devoted a single minute to spiritual life, to their improvement.

You are on earth for a very short time and when you leave you will not take your cars and houses across. All this will remain here, you will only leave with your inner acquisitions, they alone will not leave you. This is what you have not really understood yet, which is why you are continually immersed in material activities. But how will you benefit from it? When you leave the earth you will have to give up everything, and you will leave naked, poor and miserable.

Anything you can do for spiritual work, do it at least during meals. Even if it is not visible, even if nobody appreciates these things, go ahead, start collecting wealth, developing the best qualities in you. When you come back in the next incarnation, Heaven will give you the most favorable conditions for your development because you will have started doing the real work today.

Here is a page of divine Science that you must know, because even if it is not yet accepted, it is science that will triumph, that will enlighten you, that will save you.

3

FOOD, A LETTER OF LOVE OF THE CREATOR

Let's take a fruit... Without dwelling on its flavor, its fragrance, its color, let's consider this fruit filled with the rays of the sun: it is a letter written by the Creator and everything depends on how we will read this letter. If we don't know how to read it, we won't get any benefit from it, and that's a shame!

Any girl, any boy, when they receive a letter from the one they love, watch how fervently they read it, re-read it and treasure it. But the Creator's letter, we send it to the basket, it does not deserve to be read! The man is the last one who will stop to decipher this letter; the animals are more attentive than him. Yes, oxen and cows, for example, when they have not deciphered the letter well, they read it again. You laugh, you can't find this scientific explanation at all... Well, call it scientifically "ruminating", if you like, but I'm telling you that they reread the letter...

Food is a love letter sent by the Creator and must be deciphered. In my opinion, it's the most powerful, the most eloquent love letter, since it tells us: "We love you... we bring you life, strength..." Most of the time , humans swallow everything without deciphering anything from this letter where the Lord also writes: “My son, I want you to become perfect, to be like this fruit: tasty. For the moment you are harsh, sour, tough, you are not yet ready to be tasted, so you must educate yourself. Look at this fruit: if it has reached maturity, it is because it has been exposed to the sun. Like him, you must expose yourself to the sun, to the spiritual sun: it will take care of transforming in you everything that is acidic, indigestible, and it will also add beautiful colors to you. This is what the Lord tells us through food. You haven't heard it yet, but I hear it.

As we eat, food speaks to us, because food is condensed light, condensed sound. If you are always thinking elsewhere, you will not be able to hear this "voice" of light. Light is not separate from sound; the light sings, the light is a music... It is necessary to arrive to hear the music of the light; she speaks, she sings, it is the divine Word.

We can also say that nutrition is a kind of dowsing. Each being, each object emits particular radiations, and the dowser is the one who knows how to capture these radiations and interpret them. Now, food has received radiation from the entire cosmos; the sun, the stars, the four elements have left invisible but real imprints on her; they impregnated it with all kinds of particles, forces, energies. She even recorded the traces of the passage of men who walked or worked in the fields near her. She can therefore tell you her story, tell you about the sun, the stars, the angels, the Creator, reveal to you which entities have taken care day and night of infusing her with this or that property to be useful to humans, to the children of God.

Even if nature sees how sleepy and ignorant humans are, it is so generous that it says to itself: “Bah! whether they are intelligent, conscious, awake or not, I will ensure that food gives them strength so that they can maintain their life. » Like animals, all unconscious people manage to subsist thanks to food, it is obvious, but it does not make them grow spiritually, they only feel a physical well-being.

When it comes to receiving its most subtle particles from food, one must be aware, awake, full of love. At that moment the whole organism is ready to receive it in such a perfect way that the food in turn feels touched and pours out its hidden riches. If you know how to welcome someone with a lot of love, he opens up, he gives you everything; if you receive it badly, it closes. Expose a flower to light and heat, it opens, it gives off its fragrance; leave it in the cold and the dark, it closes. Food also opens or closes according to our attitude, and when it opens, it offers us its purest, most divine energies.

4

CHOICE OF FOOD

I

One day, one of my disciples who is a doctor received a phone call from a lady: her husband was in bed with a severe liver attack. "Do you think it could be from what he ate?" she asks; the day before yesterday we were invited to a wedding feast. - Oh! said our sister, and what did you eat? - Me, not much, I wasn't very hungry, but my husband ate with a very good appetite," and she begins to describe the menu. It was something incredible: sausage, sausage, ham, pâté, melon, sweetbreads with mussels, trout with almonds, rabbit with prunes, cheeses, ice cream, Saint-Honoré, fruits, all kinds of wines, champagne, coffee, liqueurs... "Do you think so, doctor," said the lady, Could something have hurt him? Many people don't relate their health to what they ate.

Yet it is with the food that he absorbs that man builds his body, and we must not therefore believe that by swallowing anything we will always be healthy, fulfilled. You have to see that there is a relationship between what you eat and the state you will be in afterwards. If we absorb all sorts of heterogeneous materials, they will pile up in the body which will no longer know how to eliminate them, and one way or another we will be sick. You always have to be careful what you let into your body.

Of course, some will quote the passage from the Gospel where Jesus says that it is not what goes into man that is important, but what comes out of him.

We must know how to interpret these words of Jesus. Is it reasonable to think that if you put rubbish somewhere, it is purities that will come out? Of course, if you are an Initiate, because of your elevation, whatever you eat, you will transform it and send it back in the form of light. Yes, but you have to be an Initiate. As for the others, if they swallow dirt, it's dirt that will come out. Watch what comes out through people's mouths or eyes because they don't know how to transform, sublimate food! They swallowed dirt, and it comes out dirt. How could they transform anything when they have no intelligence, no purity, no love, no kindness?

Jesus cannot have advised to eat and drink just anything, and moreover no Initiate will give this advice. Only if you have done great spiritual work capable of neutralizing poisons and transforming impurities into light are you free to absorb whatever you want. And by the way, the reverse is also true: until you decide to do spiritual work, even the best food will not transform you. The main thing is the power of the inner life, of thought, of feeling.

I know that those who deal with dietetics recommend certain foods and advise against others. They may be right, of course, but it is above all the way of eating that must be watched. Eat what you want, but eat it properly and in reasonable quantities, you will be healthy. I've seen lots of people on macrobiotic diets or whatever, but very often those diets didn't cure them and even weakened them. I have nothing against macrobiotics, I recognize that there is something real in it. But where I don't agree is when food is given first place. No, food is only a means. What matters most is the psychic life, the spiritual life, the food comes after.

The best food has never stopped some people from being mean, vicious, and wanting to devastate the whole world. Even vegetarianism is not omnipotent: Hitler was a vegetarian! While others who ate even meat or very bad food became saints and prophets. They had done no study, they ate what they found, lived without hygiene, but they had given preponderance to the spirit, and with the few truths they knew, an immense love for these truths and a will inflexible to achieve them, they managed to do wonders.

But back to the food we eat every day. Obviously, in the physical plane we will not find absolutely pure nourishment: we can never even really know what we are going to come across. While in the realm of feelings, thoughts, we can be very vigilant and make a choice to constantly feed ourselves with the best thoughts and feelings and reject others. Thoughts and feelings are materials from which we form our various subtle bodies, and if we build a hovel, symbolically speaking, we will not receive a visit from a prince or a high priest, but from tramps. It is we who build our etheric, astral and mental bodies, and according to the quality of these bodies, our destiny is all mapped out:

The future of man depends on how he eats. If you eat badly on the physical plane, you look bad and everyone asks you what is going on. Since the quality of food can change how you look, so can the quality of your thoughts and feelings. Some thoughts and feelings are capable of making you beautiful, and some others, unfortunately, of making you ugly. So why not be careful?

The transformation of the human being cannot be done without the acquisition of new particles of a better quality. This is why observing silence during meals is not enough, this silence we must also fill it with the highest thoughts and feelings, because then it becomes so powerful and magical that it has all the elements necessary for nourishment. of our subtle bodies. Silence is not a vacuum, there is no vacuum in nature, everything is filled with forces, with materials, with elements that become purer and purer as one rises in the higher regions, and this powerful and magical silence is a mine of riches from which we can draw.

II

The four elements (earth, water, air, fire), which correspond to the four states of matter, are contained in the food we eat every day. So, while eating, we can enter into a relationship with the Angels who preside over these four elements: the Angel of the earth, the Angel of the water, the Angel of the air, the Angel of the fire, to ask them to help us build our physical body, to make it so pure and subtle that it becomes the dwelling place of Christ, of the Living God.

Each of these Angels represents certain qualities and virtues: the Angel of the earth, stability; the Angel of Water, purity; the Angel of the air, intelligence; the Angel of fire, divine love. If, when he takes his food, man binds himself by thought to these four Angels, he receives particles of a more spiritual quality thanks to which he builds his subtle bodies, up to the body of light. When he has succeeded in building this luminous body which the scriptures call the body of glory, man becomes truly immortal.[2]. The physical body cannot last very long: it is obliged to return all the elements that compose it to the mother earth from which it came. But in his body of light, in his body of glory, man can live forever.

The body of glory is an etheric germ, a tiny germ, an electron which we all inherit and which is waiting to be formed, nourished, developed. It is a process exactly comparable to that of gestation. Just as the mother must work for months on the germ she has received from the father, adding to it the materials necessary to arrive at the formation of a living being which will perhaps be able to move the whole world, to even in the spiritual plane we have to work on the germ of the body of glory in order to develop it. As long as we don't think of it, as long as we don't take care of it, it stays there, neglected, buried, buried. Fortunately, it cannot die: it awaits the moment when we become conscious and work to develop it, to make it powerful and luminous.

This body of glory must be formed of the elements of the greatest purity, of the greatest intensity. Because only the intense vibrations of light oppose the process of illness and death, dislocation, fermentation, disintegration... When light triumphs in man, he becomes immortal. This is why it is so important that through food you learn to eat and drink light with the absolute conviction that you are thus receiving new life.

Through nutrition, you can enter into relationship with the Angels of the four elements who will become your friends and collaborate with you. So when you eat, forget your worries, your grudges, your bad thoughts, because that is what poisons the food and makes you sick. Connect with the Angels of the four elements, say: "O Angel of the earth, Angel of the water, Angel of the air, Angel of the fire, give me your qualities: stability, purity, intelligence, divine love…" and that is how you will enter into the new life.

5

VEGETARISM

Nutrition is a very broad issue, as it is not just limited to the foods and beverages we take with meals. We also feed on sounds, scents, colors. The beings of the invisible world in particular feed on odors. The habit of burning incense in churches, for example, comes from this very ancient knowledge that luminous spirits are attracted by pure odors, such as that of incense, while infernal spirits are attracted by odors nauseating. But there are not only smells: sounds and colors are also food for the invisible spirits and can be used to attract them. This is why, often, painters represent angels playing music and dressed in shimmering robes.

It is said in the Scriptures: "You are temples of the Living God". So do not defile these temples by introducing impure elements. If humans knew in which celestial workshops they were created, they would be much more attentive to the food that goes into the construction of this temple where God must come to dwell. Unfortunately, when eating meat, the majority of them look more like graveyards filled with corpses than temples.

Every creature, animal or human, is compelled to choose one food over another, and this choice is always very significant. If you want to know what the cameo food results are, go visit a zoo, watch the carnivorous animals, and you'll know right away. Moreover, it is not even necessary to go to zoos to make this observation. Human samples of all species of animals are found in existence, and even those not found in the parks, such as mammoths, dinosaurs and other prehistoric monsters! But let's be charitable and stick to zoological parks: there, you can see that large predators are formidable animals that spread extremely strong odors around them, while herbivores generally have much more peaceful manners. The food they eat does not make them violent or aggressive, while meat makes carnivores irritable. Similarly, humans who eat meat are further driven into brutal and destructive activity.

The difference between meat food and vegetarian food lies in the amount of solar rays they contain. Fruits and vegetables are so impregnated with sunlight that we can say that they are a condensation of light. When we eat a fruit or a vegetable, we therefore directly absorb sunlight, which leaves very little waste in us. While the meat is rather poor in sunlight, that is why it quickly putrefies; however, anything that putrefies quickly is harmful to health.

The harmfulness of meat has yet another cause. When the animals are taken to the slaughterhouse, they sense the danger, they feel what awaits them, and they are afraid, they panic. This fear causes a disturbance in the functioning of their glands which then secrete a poison. Nothing can eliminate this poison; it enters the organism of the man who eats meat, and this presence is obviously favorable neither to his health nor to his longevity. You will say, "Yes, but the meat is delectable. Perhaps, but you never think of anything but your pleasure, your satisfaction. It is only the pleasure of the moment that matters to you, even if you have to pay for it with the death of countless animals and with your own ruin.

Moreover, it is necessary to know that all that we absorb like food becomes inside us an antenna which collects well determined waves. This is how meat binds us to the astral world. In the lower regions of the astral world are swarming beings who devour each other like wild animals do, and so, by eating meat, we are in daily contact with the fear, the cruelty, the sensuality of animals.

He who eats meat maintains in his body an invisible link with the animal world and he would be appalled if he could see the color of his aura.

Finally, taking the lives of animals is a great responsibility; it is a transgression of the law: "Thou shalt not kill." Moreover, in Genesis, when before the fall God gave man his food, He simply said: "Behold, I give you every herb bearing seed and every tree having in it the fruit of a tree and bearing seed: this will be your food. »

By killing animals to eat them, it is not only their life that is taken away from them but also the possibilities of evolution that nature had given them in this existence. This is why, in the invisible, each man is accompanied by all the souls of the animals whose flesh he has eaten; these souls come to claim indemnities from him, saying: “You have deprived us of the possibility of evolving and instructing us, so it is now up to you to take care of our education. Although the soul of animals is not similar to that of humans, animals have a soul, and one who has eaten the flesh of an animal is obliged to bear the presence of its soul within him. This presence is manifested by states which belong to the animal world; this is why when he wants to develop his superior being, he encounters difficulties, the animal cells do not obey his desire, they have a will of their own directed against his. This explains why many manifestations of humans do not actually belong to the human kingdom but to the animal kingdom.

With regard to fish, the question presents itself differently. Fish have been placed for millions of years in very poor evolutionary conditions, as can be seen when studying the structure of their organism, their nervous system has remained very rudimentary. It is therefore allowed to eat them, which makes them evolve. In addition, there is an element in fish specially made for today's times: iodine.

The food that we take in goes into our blood, and from there it attracts the entities that correspond to it. It is said in the Gospels: “Where the corpses are, there the vultures gather”. This is true for the three worlds: physical, astral and mental. So if you want to be well in the three planes, don't attract vultures with corpses. Heaven does not manifest through people who allow themselves to be invaded by physical, astral and mental impurities.

Meat corresponds to a special element in thoughts, feelings and deeds. If, for example, you dream that you are eating meat, you must be attentive, vigilant, because it indicates that you will be exposed to certain well-defined temptations: to commit acts of violence, to let yourself be carried away by sensual desires or to have thoughts selfish and unjust. For meat represents all of this: violence on the physical plane, sensuality on the astral plane and selfishness on the mental plane.

Tradition reports that before the fall Adam had a radiant face, and all the animals loved him, respected him, obeyed him. After the fall, Adam lost this face and the animals became his enemies. If the beasts no longer have confidence in man, if the birds fly away at his approach and all creation considers him an enemy, there is a reason: it is that he has fallen from spiritual heights. where he was. It must regain its first splendor by submitting again to the laws of love and wisdom, it will then be reconciled with all the kingdoms of creation and it will be the advent of the Kingdom of God on earth.

In appearance, the war between men is due to economic or political questions, but in reality it is the result of all this slaughter that we make of animals. The law of justice is implacable: it obliges humans to pay by shedding as much blood as they have caused the animals to shed. How many millions of liters of blood spilled on the earth crying out for vengeance to Heaven! The vaporization of this blood attracts not only microbes, but billions of larvae and lesser entities from the invisible world. These are truths that we do not know and that we may not accept, but whether we accept them or not, I am obliged to reveal them to you.

We kill animals, but nature is an organism, and by killing animals, it is as if we were touching certain glands of this organism: at that moment, the functions are modified, an imbalance is created and there is no should not be surprised if some time after war breaks out among men. Yes, millions of animals have been slaughtered to eat them without knowing that, in the invisible world, they were linked to men and that these men must therefore die with them. By killing the animals, it is the men who are massacred. Everyone says that we must finally make peace reign in the world, that there must be no more war... But the war will last as long as we continue to kill animals, because by killing them, it is ourselves that we are destroying.

6

THE MORALS OF NUTRITION

Some believe that it is necessary to eat a lot to be healthy and to have strength. Not at all, it's even the opposite: by eating a lot we tire the body, we hinder and block the digestive processes, and this leads to unnecessary overloads that it is then almost impossible to eliminate. This is how all kinds of diseases appear because of this erroneous opinion that you have to eat a lot to be well.

In reality, it is hunger that prolongs life. If you always finish your meals full, sated, you will become heavy, drowsy, and you will no longer have any drive towards perfection.

Whereas if you leave the table with a slight appetite, having refused the few small bites that you still wanted, the etheric body receives an impulse to seek in the superior regions elements which will fill the void thus left. And a few minutes later, not only are you no longer hungry, but you feel lighter, more alive, more able to work, because these elements that the etheric body has gone to look for in space are precisely of a superior quality. Whereas if you eat to satiety and even beyond your needs, for the pleasure of eating as so many people do,

When you eat excessively, there is an overflow, and your etheric body, which is overworked, can no longer carry out its functions: at this time, certain lower entities of the astral plane, seeing this abundance of food, rush to take part in the feast that you are giving unconsciously. That's why a few moments later you feel a void again and you feel the desire to start eating again to fill it... And the undesirables also come back. This is how you become magnificent bait to attract and feed the thieves and the hungry of the astral plane who feast at your expense.

Of course, here too, when I talk about leaving the table hungry, I'm only talking about a very slight deprivation. If you constantly deprive yourself of a material necessary for the organism, the etheric body cannot repair these lacks. But if, on a kilo, you remove twenty grams, you feel lighter, more ready because of the etheric element which is added to the food which you have already taken.

How many times have I had this experience of eating just a little less than I was hungry! You will say to me: “But we are tempted, we want to continue! Hey, I know we're tempted! But what about reason and will? This is an opportunity to exercise them! Even in the greatest feasts, parties, receptions, you have to know how to refuse. I often refuse. Everywhere I am invited, I am presented with all kinds of dishes, and yet I have warned in advance: “Don't do anything extraordinary, give me some salad, some vegetables, some fruit. Of course, we don't take it into account, we still prepare a fantastic meal, and when we see that I only take very little of it, we are disappointed. But too bad, you had to believe me!

It's been a very long time since I understood what we lose by indulging in eating beyond our hunger; we pay for it with the loss of a subtle element much more precious than the flavor of the best dishes. You too must know how to refuse what is offered to you. If you don't refuse, you will be unable to perform important work. You will be sated, asleep somewhere, while there is spiritual work there waiting for you. You must not fall asleep, because this work must be done!

Of course, it is up to each individual to know for himself how much food is suitable for him. Everyone doesn't have the same stomach, I know that, and I've encountered a few phenomena in life. Like Tséko, for example, a brother of the Fraternity of Bulgaria:

his appetite amazed everyone, he never seemed satiated.

He was a nice boy, helpful, always smiling, always friendly. As he was extremely strong, he carried everyone's luggage. When the Fraternity went up to camp on the Moussala, he was loaded like a donkey: the sisters, especially the older ones, gave him their things to carry, and he accepted everything without retaliating, without grumbling. When we turned around on the road, we saw a whole mountain advancing. Often even, during excursions, it was he who carried on his back the samovar which the brothers and sisters used to make tea, and he carried it with the embers; the water was starting to boil, you could hear hissing, you could see smoke, and Tseko was advancing quietly, like a locomotive.

Of course, with such a good nature he was sympathetic to everyone, and everyone wanted to invite him. But wherever he went, he ate whatever was on the table. If you wanted to keep something, you shouldn't leave it in front of your eyes, because everything disappeared in this stomach, unique in the world. When we were camping in Rila there was sometimes a certain amount of food left over from meals that was put aside to be thrown away because it was already fermented. But when the nuns who took care of the kitchen went to get this food to throw it away, it had disappeared: Tséko had eaten it. But whatever he ate, he was never sick. The Master Peter Deunov, realizing what phenomenon he was dealing with, sent to him all those who had no appetite: just by watching Tséko eat, their appetite returned. Yes, it was truly a phenomenon!

And that's not all. While he had absolutely no education, he began to write poems. He believed that poetry was about finding rhymes, and so he wrote things that had no head or tail, but it rhymed! Obviously, when he read these "poems" we couldn't help laughing, it was so comical. He could clearly see that people were making fun of him, but imperturbably, with a smile - he was never offended by the mockery and criticism - he continued to read his poems to us by the fire, in the evening, in Rila. But then one day he began to write real poetry and everyone was amazed. We no longer laughed, we no longer joked.

Then he wanted to compose music, write songs. There, again, people began to laugh and joke: Tséko composer! And then, we soon noticed that the brothers and sisters who were walking in the mountains, near the Rila lakes, were humming the tunes of Tséko and singing his songs.

He was an electrician, and one day we learned with great sadness that while working on an electric pole, he had caught the current and had fallen. This is how he died. Everyone regretted him, and after fifty years, I still often think of him. In any case, I have never seen such a stomach.

But you, you are not Tséko and you must know that excess food is harmful to your health. Moreover, by eating more than is necessary, you take what was intended for others, and if many do the same, some eating too much and some not enough, there follows an imbalance in the world. Misunderstandings, revolutions, wars originate from the covetousness, greed, lack of moderation of those who accumulate wealth (food, land, objects) of which others are deprived. But the collective consciousness is not awakened to understand and foresee the remote consequences, the disturbances that these tendencies can cause.

This need to take, to absorb more than necessary, pushes beings to enslave others and even to suppress them at the slightest resistance or opposition. Even tiny, this is the starting point of great disasters. It is therefore very early that it is necessary to control, measure and regulate this instinct. If left unchecked, it can take on such gigantic proportions in all areas of existence that it will become the source of the greatest misfortunes.

This is why the disciple must learn not to go overboard in food. He must know when to stop before he is satisfied. When you don't know how to stop, you feed into yourself desires that are not natural, you become like those rich people who have the morbid need to grab everything. They are already rich, but their ambitions and lusts are so gigantic that they want to swallow up the whole world.

Jesus said that it is easier for a camel to pass through the eye of a needle than for a rich man to enter the Kingdom of God. For two thousand years this image has never been explained, and for some who did not know what argument Jesus was relying on, it was a bizarre image. In reality, Jesus was not thinking of the physical body, but of the astral body. In the rich, the body of desire, the astral body, is so swollen, dilated because of the excess of its lusts, that it becomes like an immense tumor which prevents it from passing through the door, however very wide, of the Kingdom of God.

Whereas the camel's astral body is very small because it is sober and satisfied with little. This is why he is able to traverse the deserts; where all succumb, the camel continues.

So, you see, those who have never been concerned about this question and who eat unreasonably prepare tumors in their astral bodies which will prevent them from passing through the gates of initiation. And at the same time, they get into debt, because they take what belongs to others, and this attitude is contrary to the laws of the spiritual world which require an organization, an equitable and harmonious distribution of things.

If the beings above see that you have a selfish and gross mentality, they will not accept you among them. They tell you: "Stay down in the jungle, where the beasts eat each other, that's your place", and you will complain in vain that you are gnawed, that you are pricked, as long as you do not reason according to the philosophy of the Great Universal White Brotherhood, you will suffer and the gates of Heaven will be closed to you.

It must be understood that this question of food does not stop only with physical food. For feelings and thoughts, they are the same laws. Lovers who eat without measure, until satiety, also end up having tumors in their astral body, and the door of Heaven is closed to them. The proof that Heaven has closed is that they are completely disgusted, disgusted, all their inspirations are gone, and they separate, they kill each other.

Let go of the idea that you have to eat a lot to be healthy. Because they love their children, some mothers think they are doing the right thing by force-feeding them. These are stupid mothers! Instead of force-feeding a child, we must teach him how to eat and show him the measure, make him understand that by taking for himself more than he needs, he is depriving others in one way or another, if it's not in the physical plane, it's in the astral or mental plane... Now, you have to think of others. How many of you think of sharing your wealth when you have plenty? I speak here above all for the feelings, for the thoughts. There are days when you are amazed, you feel rich, happy... Do you at that moment think a little about distributing your happiness to all those who are in suffering and desolation? No, you keep everything to yourself.

It is necessary to know how to give a little of this abundance, of this overflowing happiness and to say: “Dear brothers and sisters of the whole world, what I possess is so magnificent that I want to share it with you. Take from this happiness, take from this light! If you have the consciousness developed enough to do this, you are recorded in the records of Heaven as intelligent and loving beings. And even, what you have thus distributed will be placed on your account in the celestial banks, where you will be able to draw later when you need it. And your joy remains within you, intact, no one can take it from you because you have placed it in a safe place.

Moreover, if you knew how to observe yourself, you would notice that each time you keep a joy without wanting to share it with others, evil beings from the invisible world who are watching you send you through someone around you something that makes you lose that joy. Even when you are the happiest, something unpredictable happens that robs you of your joy. Because you didn't think of sharing it, of giving it to the Lord or to the Divine Mother, saying: "I don't know who to distribute it to, I'm so stupid! This joy is Yours, Lord, Yours, O Divine Mother; I give it to you to distribute. And the Lord and the Divine Mother distribute your joy, while part of it is deposited in the reservoirs of Heaven.

From now on try to always keep the measure when you eat because this is a question that goes much further than the only field of nutrition. Moreover, if you learned to eat with more awareness and love, even by reducing the food by half or a quarter, you would draw extraordinary energies from it. Because, in reality, the energy that a single bite can release would be able to run a train all around the earth. Yes, just one bite!

7

THE YOUNG

I

Fasting, a method of purification

When you eat, your body absorbs the elements that are useful to it and tries to get rid of those that are foreign or harmful to it. But the organism is not always able to make this discrimination, either because you have overloaded it, or because the food you eat contains too many impurities. At this time the waste accumulates in different organs, and it is the intestines that are especially clogged.

But even pure food leaves waste in us, which is why it is good from time to time to fast to allow the body to do the necessary cleaning work. Moreover, fasting is a method that nature teaches us. Observe the animals: when they are sick, they instinctively begin to fast; they go hide somewhere, find an herb that will purge them, and they heal themselves.

When you see dust on the furniture in your home, you know it needs to be removed. But when it comes to understanding that your own body also needs to be cleansed at least once a week and that the millions of workers who are the cells of your body sometimes need to be put on leave, then you don't. can't.

Some illnesses are manifested by fever, watery eyes, runny nose, skin covered with small eruptions: it is a purification. Since you don't want to purify yourself, your organs are forced to do the work for you.

Fasting is a healthy habit, and it would be good if, conditions permitting, everyone could fast every week for twenty-four hours, devoting themselves more particularly to spiritual work: bonding with luminous entities, choosing music and readings that can inspire him, purify his thoughts and feelings. Those who submit to this discipline of fasting find after a while that the materials that the body rejects by natural means lose their smell.

Suppose I am a doctor, and listen to me without being shocked by my words. If you notice that the smell of the materials you reject, as well as the smell of your perspiration, become very strong and even unpleasant, know that this is a sign that you are physically or mentally ill. You will say that these odors depend solely on the nature of the foods you ate that day. No, and even observe yourself: if for a few days you are worried, angry or jealous, your smell changes. Everything is reflected there, in the smell of the body.

Fasting for several days can also be beneficial, but again you have to find suitable conditions. It is better to arrange to fast during the holidays for example, in order to be free and to be able only to read, to walk, to meditate, to pray, to listen to music... Moreover, given that, when one fasts , it is the air that replaces the food, it is better to choose a place where you can breathe clean air.

Many will find that when they fast, they have pains in the back, or palpitations, or headaches... Since it is a special language of nature and we do not understand it, we say to ourselves "Never again will I fast. This is bad reasoning. These discomforts are nature's warnings that one day or another you will have to suffer in those same organs where you are now experiencing pain. So, if you want to know what your weak points are, fast for a few days; if you suffer then in any organ, know that it is from there that the disease can come, and take precautions.

If practiced sensibly, fasting is not dangerous and cannot harm you. The proof is that the discomforts appear especially the first two days, and then they disappear. If these discomforts came from fasting, they should increase, whereas on the contrary, peace and tranquility invade you. Nobody died from fasting for a few days once in a while, but millions of people died from overeating!

At first, fasting can seem very painful because the body is suddenly upset by this cleansing to which it was not accustomed. But one should not judge by these first effects to say that it is dangerous to fast. On the contrary, it is the people who feel discomforts who most need to fast, since these disorders come from the overabundance of waste thrown suddenly into the blood by this cleansing. Many people who rely only on appearances think that by fasting they will weaken, look bad. Again, this may be true at first, but after a few days you recover and become clear, light and pleasant to look at.

Those who want to fast must understand things differently. If they feel discomfort, they should not be frightened but continue until they stop. If they then interrupt the fast, they do like all those who, as soon as they have a fever, begin to take pills to stop it. Of course they feel better right away, but they don't know that by stopping the fever in this way, they are preparing themselves for some good illness later on.

Let your body react on its own. When the organism is congested, it reacts by trying to reject and dissolve all the waste, which is why the temperature rises. It is necessary to support this temperature, it is the proof that the cleaning is done. To help the body in its work, you can drink very hot boiled water. Drink several large bowls of it successively and the temperature will drop very quickly: all the channels will dilate and the blood will be able to circulate easily, carrying the waste towards the natural channels and the pores.

It is also very good to drink hot water when fasting. You boil it for a few minutes and then let the limestone deposit. When you wash greasy dishes in cold water, you noticed that the plates are not cleaned at all. It takes hot water to dissolve fat. It is the same for the body: hot water dissolves many elements and materials that cold water leaves intact; it then draws them out through the pores, kidneys, etc. and you feel purified, rejuvenated. You can even drink hot water every day on an empty stomach. As hot water cleans the channels, it is also an excellent remedy for arteriosclerosis and rheumatism.

First of all, it is not very pleasant to drink hot water, but little by little one feels such well-being that it becomes a real pleasure. Hot water is the most natural and harmless remedy, but maybe it's because it's too simple and too cheap that no one takes it seriously. One of our brothers was cured by hot water of a disease that his doctor had not been able to cure with other remedies. When he went to see him again, he told him how he had done it, and this doctor, who was a friend of his, confessed to him: "Yes, I know the miracles that hot water can do in many cases, but you wouldn't want me to charge a consultation to a patient to whom I would only prescribe to drink hot water! »

When you fast, the physical body feels deprived, of course, but the etheric body comes to remedy these deprivations by bringing other purer, more subtle elements. The role of the etheric body is to watch over the physical body and to recharge its reservoirs of energy. Fasting therefore gives an impulse to the etheric body which begins to work: the activity is transported elsewhere, and during this time the physical body rests.

Obviously, if you prolong the fast too long, the etheric body is overloaded with work while the physical body does nothing, which is not good either. The physical body and the etheric body are two associates, and if only one of the two works, the balance is broken. It is therefore necessary to distribute the activity harmoniously between the two.

To conclude, I will say a few words to you on how you should go about breaking a fast of several days, because you have to know that you can die if you start eating normally again right away. The first day it is advisable to take only a few cups of light broth; the next day you can eat soup with crackers, and finally on the third day you can start eating normally again, but light food and in moderate quantities. This way you will not be in any danger.

After such a fast, you experience new, subtle sensations, you have revelations and above all you feel rejuvenated, cleared, as if the materials that cluttered the body had disappeared, as if waste and impurities were burned. There are some very interesting things to study about it, but ignorance and fear prevent humans from regenerating themselves through fasting as many spiritualists and mystics used to do in the past.

II

Fasting, another way to eat

In reality, this question of fasting goes much deeper than you might imagine. What brings misfortunes to man are the impurities of his former lives. Each sin, each fault left in him like a waste, and his misfortunes are the result of all this waste which was not rejected. By fasting he gets rid of these harmful elements, the light is made and he feels lighter, happier. This is why fasting has always been advocated by religions and spiritual teachings.

Fasting is not giving up, depriving yourself, on the contrary. Fasting is primarily for food. When you deprive the physical body of nourishment, it is the other bodies (etheric, astral, mental) that begin to get to work. For in man there is a principle which defends itself, which does not want to die. If the physical body runs out of food, an alert is given, and as there are entities in the body who watch over your safety, at that time, from a higher region, these entities come to provide you with what you lack: you begin to absorb elements that are in the atmosphere and you feel nourished. And if at that moment you stop breathing for a few seconds, it is still other entities, higher up, in the astral and mental planes, who bring you food.

The esoteric tradition reports that the first man fed on fire and light. But when it descended into matter, as involution progressed. he needed thicker and thicker food until he had to eat like he does now. This is why the Initiates who know that the current way of nourishing themselves is a result of involution, try to return to the first state of humanity by learning to absorb ever more subtle elements. It is as if they were rejecting the stomach, then the lungs... This is how their thought is freed. But it is quite a long and difficult training, and even in India, very few yogis achieve such mastery of their breathing. Those who achieve this can swim in the Akasha, in the cosmic ether,

Man therefore descended from the celestial regions by a process which has been called involution.

As this descent into matter progressed, as it moved away from the primordial fire to enter the cold regions of the periphery, it took on thicker and thicker bodies...until the physical body. Exactly as we are obliged, in winter, to cover ourselves with all kinds of clothes to face the cold. To now resume the path upwards, man must undress, symbolically speaking, that is to say, get rid of everything that weighs him down. And fasting is precisely a means of rediscovering this lightness, this primordial purity.

But fasting is not just abstaining from physical food. Fasting is also giving up certain feelings, certain thoughts that weigh us down. Instead of always wanting to absorb, swallow, accumulate, you have to learn to give up, to free yourself. It is the accumulation that favors the descent. Every thought, feeling, or desire that is not of a spiritual nature sticks to us like frost on the branches of trees in winter. The spring sun has to come for the frost to melt away and for us to become ourselves again. At the moment when we will have rejected all that we have accumulated in us of uselessness, we will feel crossed, vivified by the divine breath.

Whoever wants to pile everything up in his head or in his heart has no more room in him to receive the visit of the Lord and the angels. But now, don't get me wrong. I am not saying that you should no longer use the stomach, the lungs, the intestines, no, because it is not by destroying your body that you will understand the truth. You have to keep your body with the head, the heart, the lungs, the stomach... the question is only to work to create harmony between them. This is the true meaning of fasting.

8

ON COMMUNITY

One of the essential practices of the Christian religion is communion. It was not Jesus who instituted it, it already existed for centuries, since Genesis tells how Melkhitsedek, priest of the Most High, came to meet Abraham bringing him bread and wine...

But communion should not be limited to taking a host blessed by a priest from time to time. In reality each of us must be a priest, a priest, it is a vocation that he has interiorly before the Eternal; every day he must present himself to officiate in front of his cells and give them bread and wine. If you are aware of this role, your cells will receive true communion from you, that is to say a sacred element which will help them in their work, and this joy which they will experience from having worked well, is you too who will feel it.

To understand the mystery of the Lord's Supper, nutrition must be taken as a starting point.

Of course, the breath and especially the spiritual exercises like meditation, contemplation, identification are each a form of communion, but to fully understand communion, one must begin by understanding nutrition. To meditate, to contemplate, not everyone can have conditions or even gifts for that, but everyone eats, and every day. One must therefore begin by understanding fellowship in the physical plane.

To communicate is to make an exchange: you give one thing and you receive another. You will say that in eating you only take the food. It's a mistake, you also give him something... If you don't, it's not a real communion. True communion is a divine exchange. The host brings you its blessings, but if you take it without giving it the necessary love and respect, it is not communion, it is a dishonest act. When we take, we must give. To the host you must give your respect, your love, your faith, and she, in exchange, gives you the divine elements she possesses. Those who take the host without this sacred attitude have never been able to transform themselves. It is not the object itself that acts on us, but the confidence and the love that we give to it.

To commune with the Lord, you must also give Him love, recognition, faithfulness. Not that the Lord needs what you give Him, He is so rich that He can do without it, but it is you who, by trying to give Him something from your heart, from your soul, manage to awaken certain spiritual centers, and all the divine virtues then flow in you in abundance.

But back to food. Even when you prepare your meal, you must think, by touching the food, to imbue it with your love... Speak to them, say: "You who carry the life of God, I love you, I appreciate you, I know the wealth you possess. I have a whole family to feed, millions and billions of people inside me, so be kind, give them this life. If you get used to talking to food like this, it will transform you into strength and light, because you will have known how to commune with nature itself. You will also begin to understand that true fellowship has a much broader meaning than is usually given to it by the Church.

Besides, is it smart to think that you have to wait to receive a host to truly commune with the Lord? And again, no host has ever succeeded in transforming beings. One can swallow carloads of hosts and remain the same, the same lazy person, the same thief, the same debauchee. Everything depends on the conscience... When you are aware that God has put his life in the food, when you go to eat, you are like the priest who blesses the bread and the wine, and every day, at every meal, you enter into communication with the divine life.

I am the first to understand and respect sacred things, which is why I invite you to practice them every day. For I know that a time is coming when everyone will himself become a priest before the Lord. A priest is one who understands God's creation, who loves it, who respects it. Whether he was ordained a priest or not, he is a priest, it is God Himself who consecrated him. God is above everything, He is not available to anyone, we cannot take Him by force to lock Him up in a host and distribute Him as we want. Besides, why violate the Lord when from the beginning He Himself voluntarily entered into the food? He does not like this violence and often, when we want him to be there. He is not there.

By exaggerating the importance of the host so much, we have completely neglected the question of food and forgotten that it too can bind us to God. the host, because it is all of nature, it is God Himself who prepared it from his own quintessence, so what more will a priest's blessing really bring him? ?

The Church has distorted humans so much that there is no way to make them understand now the wonders of what God has created. What they made, yes, but what God created is not interesting, they are above! Of course, if you ask the priests, they will not tell you that they consider themselves superior to God, but in practice, it is exactly as if they were putting themselves above Him. Instead of saying: "Respect life, my children, because everything is sacred, everything in nature is a talisman that God has placed for us", well no, it's only their shops that count: the hosts, the rosaries, medals, the rest does not count.

I do not belittle the role of priests, I do not belittle the importance of communion, I only want to open up new horizons for you so that you can see that communion is not only an important but indispensable act and that we need to communicate each day. By taking Communion two or three times a year, what do you think you can change about yourself? Nothing, your cells will remain the same and you will remain the same forever. To change the physical body which is so stubborn, you have to work every day on this transformation through thought, faith, love, and one day, finally, this carcass will begin to vibrate!

All the rites which have been instituted by the Church must not hide the true religion. Often we take the small glasses of a religion, a philosophy, a chapel, and all the rest is left in the shade. What's the point of belonging to a religion, if that religion is to hide the splendor of what God has created and deprive humans of the true possibilities of returning to Him?

9

THE MEANING OF BLESSING

Today most foods are poisoned with all kinds of chemicals, nothing pure or fresh can be found; fruits, vegetables are grown with harmful fertilizers and fish are caught in polluted rivers or seas... Soon we will no longer be able to live on the earth. As long as they do business and make money, most people don't care that others can die of poisoning!

However, it depends a lot on us that the food is accepted by our organism, and the prayers, the blessings before the meals serve precisely to influence it favorably and to prepare it to be well assimilated. These formulas, these prayers cannot add the least particle of life to it, because God has already put life into the food through his servants: the sun, the wind, the stars, the earth, the water. If it were possible to introduce divine life by a simple human blessing, why wouldn't we bless pieces of wood, stone, metal to eat them? By blessing a stone, a piece of wood or metal, one introduces into them a kind of life, of course, but this life cannot nourish humans; it may have another use, but it cannot be used to feed them.

"So, do you think, blessing food is useless? If, as I told you, the words and gestures of blessing envelop the food with emanations and fluids which prepare it to enter into harmony with those who must consume it; an adaptation is thus created in their subtle bodies which allows them to better receive the richness contained in this food.

This question of the blessing of food is not well understood, and the priests themselves do not know why they must bless the wine and the hosts... Those who in the past had instituted these practices were aware of their significance. magical, but now that meaning is lost. The blessing has the function of taming the food. Because it must be understood that food has its own life, and that its vibrations are therefore not always in tune with ours. So we must magnetize it, give it some particles of our being to change the movement of its particles and make it a friend. It is then that it will open up and pour into us all the riches it contains.

When two people meet, their vibrations are so different that it is not always easy for them to harmonize in order to understand each other. But time passes, there are exchanges between them, a kind of osmosis, and they begin to vibrate in unison. This also happens with food; if you eat it without prior interior preparation, it will remain a foreign matter and will not act in the same way as if you tried to enter into a relationship with it. Before eating a fruit, you have often seen me hold it for a moment in my hand: I thus transform the etheric body of the fruit by asking it to open up towards me.

You can smile at food like an animal you want to tame. Animals, plants, beings need to feel love in order to tame themselves. So it is with food... and even with medicine. For a medicine to be truly accepted by your organism and to act effectively on it, you must work on its etheric matter. Even a stone in your hand may or may not vibrate friendly to you. If you know how to make it favorable to you, it can protect you, heal you. This law is found in all areas of life. Look at what also happens with boys and girls: first of all they are strangers to each other; the girl is standing there, on her chair, upright, honest, honest, it's wonderful. But the boy offers him a drink, puts on a disc of sentimental music,

When you have to put on shoes for the first time, you feel tight, embarrassed, you find them stiff, hard, then, little by little, they become more flexible, they get used to you, so to speak. And when you settle into a new room or a new house, at first you feel out of place, the place is foreign to you. But after a while, you feel at home and you are happy to be there because this place vibrates with the life you lead.

And for food, it's curious, no one thinks there's anything to do. However, before arriving on your table, it has been lying around in all sorts of places, it has been handled, packaged, transported, so it has no connection with you, it is foreign to you. But take a fruit, hold it with respect, look at it with love: it becomes your friend, it vibrates differently. It's like a flower that opens and gives you its fragrance. The secret to making food open is to heat it, and heat is love. That's why, if you don't like this or that food, don't eat it, because then it becomes an enemy in your body. Never eat what you don't like!

Now try to do this exercise: before eating a fruit, take it in your hand, speak to it kindly, at least in thought; and so, something in that fruit will change: it will be much better disposed towards you, and when you eat it it will begin to work for you.

Learn to awaken all the powers that have been dormant within you through centuries of inertia and stagnation. Concentrate, meditate, pray, do exercises. Always have the desire to add something more to your existence, something purer and more subtle.

10

THE WORK OF THE MIND ON THE MATTER

I

Solar energy is condensed in the fruits and vegetables that we use as food. It is thus necessary to know how to extract this energy and to send it in all the centers in us which will ensure the distribution of it. But this is only possible through a work of thought. Only conscious thought focused on food is able to open it to release the trapped energy. In reality, this is a process identical to that observed in a nuclear power station. If we really knew how to eat, just a few mouthfuls could be enough... we would draw enough energy to move the whole universe.

This fission process does not occur only in the stomach, but also in the lungs and in the brain. You say, "In the brain? Yes, in his meditations, in his ecstasies, an Initiate constantly sends through space waves, currents, flames. Where does he get this energy from? From his brain. And yet if we weigh it, its mass has remained the same. The disintegration of some particles of matter takes place in the brain and it is from this disintegration that the psychic energy comes which will work in the whole world.

Contemporary science has discovered the splitting of the atom; these are processes that the Initiates have known for millennia, only they did not reveal them because they saw the danger in them; they knew that man, not yet mastering his instincts, would use his discoveries to annihilate everything, and that is what is happening. But in the future, when more evolved humans will have access to the great mysteries of nature, they will know how to draw energies from the ocean, the air, minerals, trees, etc... and they will be capable of prodigious achievements.

For now, at least understand what energies you can draw from food by involving thought in the processes of nutrition. Nutrition is a war between the human organism and the foods that are destined to become assimilable matter, and what is not assimilable is rejected. To be properly absorbed, food must be torn apart, destroyed, because the organism is obliged to destroy in order to be able to build. This is done automatically, outside of our consciousness, but by thought we can also act on food to open it and draw from it all the energies that will allow us to undertake our material tasks and our spiritual work more easily. .

II

Man eats, all creatures eat, but why? If you ask anyone, they'll tell you they eat to build strength. Yes, but isn't there another reason? Everything we do has more than one reason, one goal, and if we eat, it's not just to keep us alive.

Take the example of worms: they swallow the earth and then reject it; by thus making it pass through them, they work it, they add an element to it which makes it more fertile. With food man does the same. Since he is a being endowed with life, feeling and thought, he belongs to a degree of evolution much higher than that of the matter he absorbs, which is why in passing through him, matter is transformed, animated, refined, spiritualized.

All beings feed: plants, animals, men... and by feeding, they cause matter to evolve, they give it elements that it does not possess... as if it were a duty for each kingdom of nature to feed on the lower kingdoms in order to make them evolve. Above us, certain more advanced beings also take care of digesting us in order to transform us. Yes, in another form, that's exactly what happens. All of life is an uninterrupted exchange between the inorganic world and the organic world, between the material world and the spiritual world.

These exchanges are found all over the world. Why do intelligent people want to deal with the ignorant to educate them? Why do those who are good, generous, virtuous deal with delinquents and criminals? And the strong who help the weak... the rich who help the poor... For there to be an evolution, it is necessary that exchanges take place between the two opposite poles. And that's also the reason we eat. The Cosmic Intelligence could no doubt have found other means, but this is the one it chose: it decided that, in order to evolve, each creature would have to be absorbed by the creatures of the kingdom which is superior to it.

I gave you the example of the worms: when they reject the earth that they have absorbed, it is already more elaborate, it is impregnated with a more living element that the worms have communicated to it. And if the worms have been given this task of passing through them all the earth to improve it, why not humans? So you see, humans and worms are collaborators! They have the same task, although they ignore each other. They signed contracts above, before descending, the worms in one form and the humans in another, committing themselves to work on matter to vivify it. Signing contracts... it makes you laugh... Well, laugh, so much the better, it will do you good.

Moreover, when the matter that man possesses, when the particles of his body leave after death to join the four elements: earth, water, air, fire, they are more intelligent, more alive, more expressive, and they will serve for other forms, other creations of superior quality. But if these particles are degraded because of the animal or criminal existence that man has led, they will only be used for gross creations. Look how far human responsibility goes.

Yes, man is responsible for what he leaves of himself after his departure, for all the particles of his body that he has impregnated with light, love, goodness, purity, or, on the contrary, with criminal vibes; he continues to be responsible, even after his death. Obviously on earth, it's different: even if he has committed crimes or left debts, once dead, we can no longer prosecute him, because where to find him to punish him? On earth, death fixes many things, but on the other side death fixes nothing and man continues to be prosecuted for all the bad things he left behind: thoughts, feelings, acts. ... These are truths that most ignore; they do not know how far their responsibility goes. Yet the consciousness of responsibility is the highest consciousness that exists.

Eating, drinking, breathing, working, are all activities by which we transform matter to try to give it what we have, that is to say more life, more love, more intelligence. Plants feed on minerals, animals feed on plants, humans feed on animals. And who eats humans? This is a question we haven't asked ourselves...

In reality, two kinds of creatures feed on humans. Look: among humans, some eat the flesh of animals and others are satisfied with their products: eggs, milk... The entities of the invisible world do not come to eat the flesh of humans, but their emanations, their thoughts, their feelings, and depending on whether they have good or bad thoughts, good or bad feelings, men offer food to the Angels or to the lower spirits. Obviously, it is necessary to understand in what form this is done... And the Angels, themselves, serve as food for the Archangels, the Archangels for the Principalities... and so on, up to the Seraphim whose emanations nourish the Lord.

From time immemorial the Initiates, who possessed a science that they could not teach the crowd, have used images that must be interpreted. It is said in the Bible that the Lord delights in the smell of burnt offerings. You think if the nostrils of the Lord can really take pleasure in sniffing the smell of fat from roasted animals!... It was an image to show that the spiritual emanations of beings (burnt offerings were offered to God in sacrifice) can food to higher entities, up to the Lord...

Because God also feeds. Since we are created in his image and we eat, it is because God must also eat. Obviously it does not happen as for us, with a mouth, teeth, stomach, intestines - we cannot even have an idea of how the Lord feeds himself, so much in Him is pure and sublime - but He feeds. Otherwise, why write nonsense in the Bible - which God inhaled with delight the odor of the victims - if there was not behind these words a deeper truth?

Man's task is to make matter pass through his body to animate it. And that's why he eats. Have you calculated all that a man eats during his life?... And as for millions of years the whole of humanity has been doing the same thing, this constantly produces changes everywhere, the earth is therefore no longer the same. All the more so since there are certain very generous, very conscientious people who fulfill their task with such ardor that they eat lavish meals five or six times a day to contribute to the transformation of matter. These are people we must support and reward! But yes, look, they are doing a magnificent job: how many pigs, turkeys, chickens and rabbits are disappearing every day thanks to them! It's that they want to improve the creation, we must never forget that! While these little vegetarians there, nibbling on a few salads, they do not deserve a pedestal to be set up for them: they do not transform matter as abundantly as all these ogres and ogresses!...

In reality, the question is not only to make matter pass through his stomach, but also through his lungs, his heart, his brain... The life that we receive does not remain in us, it leaves. goes, it flows, and it is constantly another life that we receive, always new, always fresh. It is therefore not only by eating that we can improve matter, but by all our actions: by looking, by walking, by working... Yes, that is how far the understanding of nutrition must go. To be useful to all creation, to bring, we too, to the whole world a divine element, we must learn to live a perfect life, in order to permeate everything around us luminously. And by having this ideal of making everything more alive, more

luminous, more beautiful, it is
ourselves who transform ourselves,

11

THE LAW OF EXCHANGES

I

It is amazing to see that humans, who claim to fathom the mysteries of creation, neglect to look into such important processes as nutrition, in which God has put all his wisdom and his love. If we study the laws of nutrition, we find that they are found everywhere in the universe, since these are the laws that govern the exchanges between the sun and the planets, and that they are valid for all areas, and in particular that of love. Yes, even the laws of conception, of gestation are identical to those of nutrition.

In everything we eat, fish, fruit, vegetables, or even cheese, there is something to remove: a bone, a skin, a crust... And if there is nothing to remove, at least wipe or wash the food. Therefore, before eating, one must take precautions so as not to injure the palate, break one's teeth or damage one's stomach. So why don't we do the same in life? Before bonding with someone, before accepting him into his heart, into his soul, why imagine that he is already ready to be absorbed and digested? You will say: “But it is love! Yes, I understand, it's love, but that love is blind, it's not true love. True love is enlightened, it is not at odds with wisdom.

People bond, kiss, make exchanges, without getting ready, or washing, or getting rid of the filth they have picked up in their hearts and in their souls through the chimneys of life. An Initiate acts differently: when he sees a person appearing in front of him, he regards it as a “juicy fruit”, of course, but a fruit that he will have to wash or peel before “eating” it.

This is the difference that exists between Initiates and ordinary men without light, without wisdom, without knowledge: the way in which they make exchanges and associations. Ordinary people are like cats who swallow mice with their skin and intestines, and after they complain, they cry out: “Ah, how unhappy I am with my wife! Or else: "Ah, what a husband I fell on!" But why do they have the cat mentality? Why did they rush to eat this woman or this man, that is to say, why did they frequent him, why did they accept without thinking his feelings, his thoughts, his breathing, his aura?

Now analyze yourself and revise your existence... You will find that up to now you have only dwelled on external details, without going deeper to see what were the desires, feelings, thoughts or ideals of the creatures to which you wanted to bond. The Initiates are very difficult, and they are right; they have understood the lesson that nature gives us every day through nutrition, they know that we must act in the same way in psychic life. Every day we know that we have to peel, clean, eliminate, but in the psychic field we have not yet understood the lesson that nature gives us. Look, even a mother who adores her child and who will do anything for him, if he comes to kiss him after playing in the mud, she sends him first to wash up, and then she kisses him.

You take your meals three times a day, you sort the food before eating it, but you link your existence to that of the first comer, without knowing it, at the risk of being poisoned all your life. Only the Lord you must love before you know Him. Whereas humans, you have to know them before loving them, that is to say before "eating" them, inviting them into your sanctuary. If we don't love God first, we will never know Him. And for a great Master, it's the same law: you will never know him and he will remain closed to you if you don't start by loving him.

Obviously, the question now is how to love it. Most like a Master like a lake in which we go to wash ourselves, leaving all our dirt behind. They don't think that others will come to drink in this lake... and then, what will they drink? Most of those who come to have an interview with a Master pour on him all that they have picked up that is unclean during their existence, and it is the Master who must then wash himself to reject these impurities or else transform them, which which is extra work for him! So if even a Master is forced to cleanse himself, how much more so are other men! Ah, but they don't need to clean up...they've been around all the devils, and they don't even notice they're covered in splatter.

But let's put that aside and get back to the lesson we can learn from nutrition every day. Each being is like a fruit or another food of which only the digestible and tasty part must be kept. God has placed a spark in every being, and it is only with this spark that you must seek to make contact. If you don't just look at the outer side, you can even find that spark in animals, plants, stones. All creatures have this buried spark, even criminals, and if you know how to awaken it, rekindle it within them, you can address it, commune with it.

An Initiate does not want to relate to the lower nature of humans, their personality. He knows that in the cellars of a house there are rats, mold, and it is better to go up to the upper floors. Unlike ordinary people who are only interested in the faults of others and even meet to talk about them, in all the beings he meets, an Initiate seeks the buried divine spark to link it to the Heavenly Father, to the Mother Divine... He thus works on them, and one day the light comes to visit these beings. This is how an Initiate works on his disciples: he takes care of this divine spark which begins to awaken and this is why the disciple loves his Master, because a Master addresses himself to what is better in him.

And you too, when you meet a human being, remember to discover that hidden spark within him, his Higher Self, to help him make a connection with the Lord. This is the most evolved, the highest form of love: knowing how to bind only to the divine spark in each creature to nourish it, to strengthen it. There you don't have to be suspicious, or waste time studying it before you love it, because that spark is pure... If it's about personality, it's better to know it before accepting it, but immediately accept the divine spark that shines in every being.

II

Men and women can be compared to fruits, I told you... When you have relations with them, when you look at them, talk to them, listen to them, it is as if you were taste them. But what do you do most of the time? You look at their clothes, their jewelry, their face, you look no further for the life that is there, hidden, the spirit, the soul. However, it is she who should interest you. No, we stop on the outer side and say: "Ah, this young girl, if only I could sleep with her! and we take pictures... But what did we see? In the desire to satisfy himself, to have fun, we only saw the outward appearance: his legs, his chest, his gently upturned little nose.

An Initiate also wants to be nourished, but he seeks divine life. And when he finds fruit or flowers, that is to say human beings who carry this life within them, he does not throw himself on them to devour them, he is content to admire their colors, their shapes, breathe in their perfume, their emanations, and he leaves happy, because these fruits and these flowers have enabled him to approach Heaven.

If you can understand nutrition, you can solve all problems, including the sexual problem. Yes, all those who have decided not to feed themselves in this area, that is to say, who run away from men or women under the pretext of being chaste and pure, die spiritually, and sometimes even physically. The question is therefore to “eat”, but you have to know what to eat and how to eat.

The secret is to learn how to eat with homeopathic doses, that is to say by watching, listening, breathing. We must not stop eating under the pretext of becoming a saint and knowing the Lord, because at that moment we do not know the Lord or anything at all, and even life goes away, we are there, without momentum, without inspiration, without joy. Holiness is nutrition, my dear brothers and sisters, this is what the Initiates have understood; but instead of taking heavy, heavy, impure food, they eat everything that is divine. In the field of sexuality, humans always go to extremes:

either they allow themselves to die of hunger, or they rush wildly to eat until indigestion.

You will find the solution when you begin to study nutrition and the different ways of nourishing yourself in all the planes. You will understand that we cannot live without eating, and that even the angels, even the Lord are obliged to eat. The Lord is nourished by the most subtle quintessences of the trees he has planted: his creatures. The Lord eats, yes, and He is well, I assure you! He is well, because he knows how to eat properly, He absorbs no impurity; all that is impure, He leaves it to others to transform before bringing it to Him.

You wonder how you can tell if someone is eating well or not... And how do you tell if a man is a tramp who looks for his food in the garbage cans, or a prince whose table is covered every day with the most succulent dishes?... It is the same in the spiritual plane. The Initiates look different from ordinary men, because they are well "nourished", while the others eat anything.

For me, there is a criterion: when I see someone who has no light on his face, I know he is undernourished. You will say: "Yes, but he goes to church, he gives money to the poor, he lowers his eyes when he meets a woman..." It is possible, but I see that inside he is eating a stale food. Whereas if I meet a radiant being, whatever people tell me about him, I think: "That one, he has a secret and I want to learn this secret, because it is a source that gushes forth!" Someone will say, "But I saw him looking at women on the beach!" It doesn't matter, what's important is what he's looking for and what he sees.

If a man rises to Divinity by marveling at the beauty of women, why do you want to prevent him? “But a pure man, a saint, never does that, you have to stick to the old rules! - Ah good, but then, you, with all your purity and your holiness, why are you weak, dull, without momentum or inspiration? How is it that your holiness has brought you nothing? And how is it that his so-called wantonness brought him Heaven and light? So there is also something to study here. You see that people do not know how to think or reason.

Exchanges are the basis of life: exchanges with food, water, air, human beings, but also with all the creatures of the universe, with angels, with God. Exchanges are not just about food, eating, drinking. Or, yes, it's eating and drinking, but in all areas, not just in the physical plane. So when I say nutrition should be in the first place, I'm talking about nutrition in all planes, the exchanges we have to make with the different regions of the universe to feed everything in us from our physical body to to our most subtle bodies. If I often insist on the need to purify oneself both physically and psychically, it is because purity restores communications,

Prayer, meditation, contemplation, ecstasies are also nutrition, the best, the most sublime, because there you taste celestial nourishment, ambrosia. All religions speak of a potion of immortality that the alchemists have called the elixir of immortal life. And it is true that one can find this elixir in the physical plane, but on the condition of seeking it there in the highest regions, the purest.

When we go to contemplate the sunrise, it is precisely to drink this ambrosia that the sun distributes everywhere and from which the rocks, plants, animals, humans, all of creation, collect particles. Moreover, plants are smarter than humans: every day, they bind themselves to the sun in order to bear fruit. While humans will sleep until noon, or else they will go to see the sunset. Instead of looking at what rises, what grows and flourishes, they prefer to look at what descends, what falls, dies and fades away. And since there is a law according to which one ends up resembling what one looks at, what one loves, then they too, inside, begin to weaken, to sink.

The meaning of life is hidden in nutrition; you will discover it if you take care to introduce into yourselves only pure, luminous particles, celestial, eternal quintessences. These particles, you will find them in the sun. This is why, each morning, concentrate on the sun and try to breathe, to absorb these quintessences which it propagates. You will see how your health will improve, your intelligence brighten, your heart rejoice and your will grow strong.

You'll say that for years you've been going to sunrise and you haven't felt anything yet... It's because you don't know how to look at it. It's the way you do things, the intensity of your love, of your thought that gets results, not the time you put into it. If today you feel so invigorated, fulfilled, it is quite simply because you have taken a few sips from this inexhaustible source that is the sun. Is it so hard to understand?

The sun is food, my dear brothers and sisters, never forget it, and the best food. Why limit yourself to the elements of earth, water and air? You have to learn to eat with fire, with light. And that's what we do at sunrise. When Zoroaster asked Ahura Mazda what the first man ate, Ahura Mazda replied, “He ate fire and he drank light. That is to say, the rays and the life of the sun thanks to which one can understand all the mysteries of the universe.

III

And now, if I tell you that the laws of nutrition are the same as those of conception, again you will be surprised, because you see no correspondence between the two. In reality, the correspondence exists: from the moment you eat, you create the conditions for the birth of thoughts, feelings, acts. If you don't eat, what can you do? Just as the state of the father and mother during conception determines the destiny of the child to be born, so the state in which you eat will determine the nature of your physical and mental activity... At each bite you take there occurs a conception. So, what state are you in as you make this design?

Food is the living germ which must produce a child, that is to say thoughts, feelings, acts. What forces will emerge from this union? Will these children be malformed, weak, weak, because of the ignorance of the father and the mother? The father is you, since you give the food; the mother is your physical body. If the father and mother are not attentive, intelligent, reasonable, the results will be catastrophic.

When you have eaten in a state of confusion, anger or discontent, and then you go to work, you feel within you a feverishness, disordered vibrations which are transmitted to everything you do. Even if you try to give the impression of calm, in control, there is something restless and tense about you. Whereas if you have eaten in a harmonious state, this state will be maintained: even if all day long you are obliged to run to the right and to the left, you feel within you a peace that your activity cannot destroy.

So don't go to the table with worries, put them aside, you will take them back later if you really want to, and because you will have eaten in a good state, you will solve your problems more easily. I repeat, meals are the occasion for the best spiritual exercises. So start by clearing your mind first of all that can keep you from eating in conditions of peace and harmony. And if you can't do it right away, wait until you have managed to calm down; otherwise you will poison the food, and then you will be in a chaotic state as a result of your faulty way of eating.

But how to make humans understand the importance of the state in which they take their meals, when certain couples, even at the moment when they create a child - an act so heavy with consequences - are in the process of hating each other? They do not know what abominations they are introducing into the child who will be born, and later this child will suffer and poison those around him.

Nutrition is a form of conception, and love is a form of nutrition. Know that Heaven holds you accountable for what you put into your partner's soul and heart. The rest doesn't matter so much. If you kiss your loved one when you're unhappy, depressed, only to finally feel relieved, as often happens, well, that's criminal, because you gave him all your dirt. It was not necessary to choose this moment. Love whoever you want, kiss whoever you want, but not before you have developed the best of your heart and your soul, the brightest part of you, to give to the being you love. Only then will Heaven not condemn you. If humans see you, maybe they will condemn you, but Heaven applauds you.

After nine months spent in its mother's womb, when the child is born, its umbilical cord is cut, and it then feeds independently.

However, even out of the womb of his mother, the human being is still in the womb of another mother, Nature, and he is nourished by another umbilical cord, the solar plexus. In India, in China, in Japan, there are very old techniques for learning to nourish oneself through the solar plexus. You would like to know them... but what would you do when you are not yet able to take your meals according to the rules I have given you?

How not to be seized with admiration in front of this divine Intelligence which arranged everything so marvelously? We eat a few fruits, and now this food, once digested and assimilated, contributes to the life of the whole organism. What is this Intelligence which is able to bring to each organ of our body what it needs so that we can continue to live? Thanks to this food we will continue to see, to hear, to breathe, to taste, to touch, to speak, to sing, to walk. And also our hair, our nails, our teeth, our skin, etc... will receive their nourishment to continue to develop.

Yes, how not to be seized with admiration before this Intelligence? From now on you must think more of her, try to discover her, to relate to her, to thank her and even, from time to time, ask her permission to be present at the work that is being done in all nature. Yes, because the day you are ready, she can accept you in her innumerable sites to show you how she works, whether in yourself or in the bowels of the earth, where minerals, metals, the crystals, the gemstones... and that's when you make the real discoveries.

What do you think is the origin of initiatory science? It was given to us by beings who had developed certain faculties of duplication which enabled them to go and visit the interior of the earth and the oceans as well as the other planets, and even the sun where they could observe a whole life unimaginable to humans: a land populated by the most evolved, luminous creatures. For what the Psalms call "Aretz ha Haïm: the Land of the Living" is the sun.

So, these so evolved spirits who visited all the regions of the universe populated by innumerable creatures left us initiatory Science as a heritage, and it is this Science that I am presenting to you now. To reassure you I will tell you that I still know very little about it, but I hope that one day I will know more. And above all, please don't prevent me from hoping for it!

www.ingramcontent.com/pod-product-compliance
Lightning Source LLC
LaVergne TN
LVHW012059160826
845678LV00014B/2879

* 9 7 9 8 8 4 6 3 7 6 2 6 7 *